POWER POSES

YOUR EMPOWERING PRACTICE GUIDE

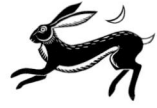

Leaping Hare Press

CONTENTS

POWER POSING

The world has a confidence crisis. Anxiety levels are surging, while reported levels of self-esteem are dropping, meaning millions of us lack the self-belief to fulfil our dreams. We could blame this sad fact on many things, ranging from how difficult events have changed our psychology and rattled our sense of self, to how we continuously see and compare ourselves to the curated 'perfection' we see online.

While there are mind-focused solutions – like therapy and mindfulness – to overcome these challenges, finding our most confident selves also involves changing how we treat and hold our physical bodies.

For a long time, we've known that our stance sends messages to other people about our power, confidence and emotions. Our physical selves are so powerful that how we use them is dubbed our 'body language', a whole separate form of communication that's just as important as the words we say. However, our body language doesn't only communicate our feelings and beliefs to others; it also tells our own minds stories about who we are.

PHYSICAL SHIFTS

When a primate has to take over as the leader of its pack, studies have found that its body adapts in order to take charge. There's a spike in testosterone, the hormone associated with dominance, and a drop in the stress hormone cortisol, making them assertive yet calm – the perfect traits for a leader.

Leader of this subject, social psychologist Dr Amy Cuddy, wanted to know if these characteristics could be reverse-engineered. That is, rather than our hormones dictating how we handle situations, could *acting* dominant make us dominant?

Her lab at Harvard Business School investigated this, and found that just two minutes of holding dominant postures was long enough for people to report feeling more powerful and less stressed, and for hormonal changes to occur as well.

These two-minute poses can be an invaluable way to help ourselves feel confident and calm under pressure. If you have a meeting where you need to prove who's boss, or want to ask for a pay rise, standing in a powerful way will help you feel more able to convince them of your brilliance.

SPIRITUAL CONNECTION

Power posing can be a long-term way to nurture your inner belief in yourself, too. For centuries, yoga has been used to form a better connection with the self, leaving practitioners more grounded and surer of their abilities.

While research shows that expansive, standing yoga poses can increase energy and improve self-perceived levels of power, yoga itself teaches us that we all have an internal fire to tap into. Specifically, our third chakra, known as the manipura or navel chakra, is directly linked to our sense of self, self-esteem and personal identity.

Yoga can also teach us that there is strength in surrender. Learning to hold still in vulnerable poses or dig deep to find balance in unstable positions can develop our ability to get over difficult moments off the mat.

As with any physical practice, ensure you are fit and well enough to perform the moves described before taking part. Some yoga poses, especially balancing and inversions, may not be suitable for everyone. Some of these poses are taken from ancient and traditional practices, so please also perform them with respect for their lineage.

HOW TO USE THESE CARDS

These cards are designed to be a tool you can turn to for guidance. Pick a card for when you need a simple pose to boost your inner power, or work through the deck to learn more about postures that will keep you calm and confident in future.

The cards are divided into three categories:

✴ **PREPARATION POSES**
These are poses you can use before stressful or big events, when you want to feel confident and assert your power. They are bigger, more visible practices than you may want to do in front of others.

✴ **POWER POSES**
These power postures can be used during events to maintain your cool. Not only do they work to indicate your confidence to others, but also to yourself.

✴ **FLOW POSES** These are poses for long-term grounding, confidence and openness. They're best used as part of a daily practice, grounded in the teachings of yoga, for a settled mind.

PREPARATION POSES

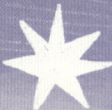

Whether you're about to tackle a personal challenge like running your first marathon, facing a professional milestone or if you just want to start the day strong, these poses can prepare you for an assured rest of your day. They're simple enough for beginners and powerful enough for regular somatic practitioners.

PRIDE POSE

Picture an athlete crossing the finish line as they've taken gold, their arms extended overhead with palms open towards the sky. This victory pose is shown to be an intuitive physical celebration, with research showing that blind athletes also take this position when celebrating their wins despite never seeing it before. Scientists suggest this might be because making ourselves bigger shows dominance, which is more likely to lead to success, so we have evolved to associate wide postures with winning. Putting yourself into the physical position of a medalist is a great way to set your mindset ahead of a big event – whether you're racing the 400-metre race at the Olympics, presenting in front of your office or simply preparing for a new day.

UPWARD SALUTE

Stretching your hands overhead is a natural way to decompress your body after lying in bed all night or having spent a day folded over your desk. This reaching pose – known in yoga as Urdhva Hastasana – is the basis of sun salutations, a sequence designed to energize the body for any upcoming yoga practice as well as the day ahead. Performed alone, the pose also has benefits, including stretching your spine, reducing discomfort to rid yourself of distractions and deepening your breath to ease you into a calmer state. It's also a grounding pose designed to bring your awareness back to yourself and nature – sun salutations were developed as a ritual to thank the sun for giving life.

SHAKE

You may think of involuntary shaking as a sign of stress or fear in humans and animals. But the purpose of those shakes is actually to get rid of the excess cortisol and adrenaline that is produced as part of your fear response. You can get a similar effect by intentionally shaking, which helps to release the stress from your body. For a longer practice, look to trauma-releasing exercise (TRE) therapy, designed by Dr David Berceli. But in the meantime, you can also simply 'shake' out nerves for a few minutes to bring out your most confident self.

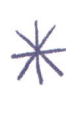

THE SERENA

Tennis player Serena Williams is one of the most powerful sportspeople of all time. Think about her posture and pose when she's about to serve on centre court: her body is open, her gaze is fixed and she exudes effortless confidence. This isn't an accident: she allegedly uses power posing as a technique to calm her mind and assert dominance on the court. While you might not be prepping for your ball toss at Wimbledon, holding a Serena-esque pose is a brilliant way to conjure the mental strength of one of tennis's best servers.

INNER STRENGTH STANCE

Although showcasing your muscles might feel like the reserve of bodybuilders, it's not just for vanity. Research suggests that flexing your muscles can actually improve their strength – in one study, by as much as 50 per cent. Given that a powerful body can create a powerful mind, activating your muscles won't just bolster your physical strength, but it will also build your mental resilience. Flexing doesn't just show you how strong you are, it also lets your body prove it.

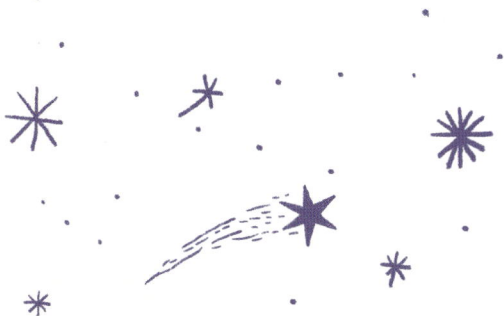

THE SELF-HOLD

This posture was designed by Dr Peter Levine, a psychologist specializing in somatic practice for trauma. He believes that the body is a container for feelings and that bringing awareness to this can stop strong emotions – like nerves and stress – from being too overwhelming. The strategic hand placement brings awareness to your heart, helping relax negative feelings, making it a perfect tool for when you need to keep calm during big moments.

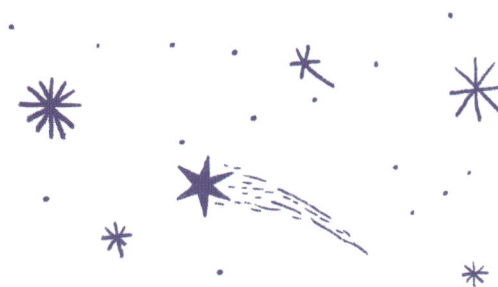

CHILD'S POSE

Known as one of the most grounding yoga poses, as so much of the body is being supported by the floor, Balasana, also known as child's pose, isn't necessarily a demonstration of power, but instead has an unrivalled ability to build confidence and calm. It's typically used as a moment of stillness in yoga flows, helping you recentre and come back to your body and breath. The same grounding can be useful during pre-event stress.

STANDING THINKER POSE

It's believed that hips hold on to negative emotions, and that opening the hips can boost confidence by removing stress from the body. This pose also has the bonus side effect of making the body physically bigger and stimulating all the benefits of a power pose. You've likely seen plenty of people take this cool, dominant position with a raised leg and casual lean before, signalling their ease in conversations and situations. Spending a moment here can trigger this self-belief in yourself, too.

LIGHTNING BOLT POSE

Like pride pose, the lightning bolt pose is another favourite of athletes – specifically runner Usain Bolt. He uses the pose – which originated as a dancehall move – to hype up the audience around him and celebrate himself after achieving world records. You can use this pose to lighten your mood and ignite creative sparks, taking the seriousness and worry out of whatever you're set to do.

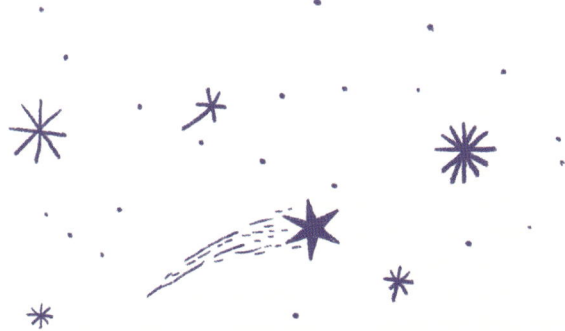

MA BU

Karate and kung fu pros exude an invincibility that not only comes from their large-and-in-charge physical positions, but also their hyper-focus and body control. While a two-minute martial arts hold may not give you the same mental focus as a full karate session, it can get you in the mindset of a fighter who is ready to take charge. It will also take some inner power to not let aching muscles pull you out of this pose.

INNER TEACHER

In yoga, saying 'namaste' is as much a physical act as it is a verbal one. It translates to 'I bow to you', and is accompanied by the prayer gesture. It isn't just an acknowledgement of respect for other people though. The bowing and prayer symbols can be just as much an acknowledgement of the divinity in yourself. When pressing your thumbs to your forehead, known as your third eye or sixth chakra, it also deepens the connection to your higher knowledge and intuition.

DYNAMIC FORWARD FOLD

Inversions have many benefits in yoga, including improving energy and circulation, but one of the biggest perks is their ability to change your perspective by quite literally flipping things upside down. Take a moment here in Uttanasana, also known as forward fold, to reframe your worry as gratefulness and turn any fear into excitement. Given this energizing pose is also associated with improved self-esteem, that viewpoint change will be easier than it sounds.

STAR POSE

When you need to shine brightly, take star pose. This simple yet harmonizing posture is designed to support the flow of energy and breath through the body, opening up from every point for balance and calm. It's a great pose to calm pre-event jitters while also helping you step into your power by opening the body, taking up space and grounding. Saluting to the sky can also help you feel inspired by the creativity of the universe.

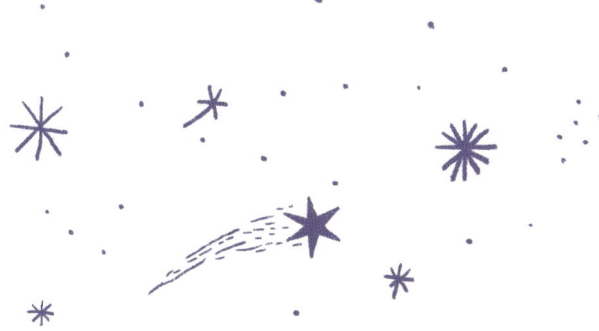

PRAYER POSE WITH VISUALIZATION

Sportspeople often visualize themselves in the final match of their competition, shooting the ball and scoring the point, or crossing the finish line with other racers dragging behind. 'Seeing' yourself succeed can be a powerful way to boost self-belief, while also training the mental muscle, which can lead to more success. Despite sitting in prayer pose, this practice isn't about 'asking' a God or divinity to create this outcome. It's about committing to your own power.

ENERGIZING BREATH

While calming breath is a popular practice, we can also use our inhales and exhales to upregulate our nervous system, improving focus, clarity and energy. This technique, also known as the 5-3-3 breath, was invented by basketball coach Dominique Williams as a way to focus athletes before a game. It uses sharp, inhale-focused breathing to stimulate the nervous system and encourage alertness. Try it before a big moment that requires you to perform at your best.

POWER POSES

Have you ever felt confidence drain
from your body the second you start
talking or getting started on your
goals? Sometimes, no matter how
prepped we are, we need an
in-the-moment boost, and
these poses can help. Draw
a card, memorize the posture
and do it the next time you
need a boost of confidence.

WONDER WOMAN

The Wonder Woman stance has become a symbol of power. It's easy to see why: the wide arms, open chest and grounded feet tick all the boxes of a power pose, giving an expansive, large presence that exudes confidence. First seen on Lynda Carter, who played Wonder Woman in the original TV series in 1975, and a favourite of superstar Beyoncé Knowles, you can adopt this pose to channel high-status energy when you're asking a colleague for a favour, talking to someone at a party or speaking publicly.

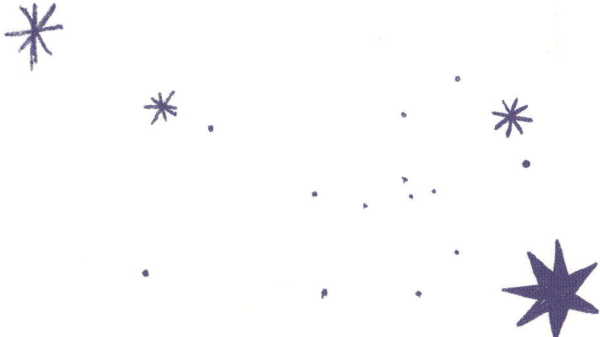

EMPOWERED POSE

This position is one of the best to boost your self-esteem and assert power in a room. Positioning yourself above others will signal your dominance to your own mind, while leaning forwards into conversation shows others you're engaged with discussions, in control of the conversation and a trustworthy leader. It's a great position to take when closing a deal or trying to come out on top of negotiations.

CONFIDENCE POSE

Taking the legs wide in this pose will stretch the hips to let go of tension while subtly taking up space. It also looks casual and cool, which can work to de-escalate tense situations. Don't disrupt others' space while doing this pose. Instead, do it sat in your own chair and in a space with plenty of room and no risk of anyone feeling your knees graze theirs. Use this pose to feel the mental benefit of physically taking up space.

MOUNTAIN POSE

Known in yoga as Tadasana, mountain pose is a move you can practise without raising eyebrows. As the name suggests, this posture is all about sturdiness and grounding while unfurling the body for inner and outer strength. Yoga is as much about mindset as it is the physical shapes, so this pose is best used in conjunction with slow, meditative breathing and mental focus to help you project stability.

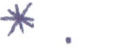

CEO POSE

This pose is great for exuding total ease. It's not a subtle pose, which helps indicate that you are totally cool and in control, and is best for casual meetings or situations in which you genuinely are in charge (hence why it's so often seen on CEOs or leaders). This big posture is a grandiose way to signal your power to others and to yourself.

THE STEEPLE

Your hand gestures make a huge difference to your display of power. Flailing or awkwardly placed hands can show anxiety, and your brain constantly thinking about what to do with your extremities can be a big distraction. Instead, take the steeple pose, a gesture used by world leaders and other high-powered people to show expertise and focus. You can do it seated or standing, when talking or listening, but you'll always have a solution to the worry about what to do with your hands.

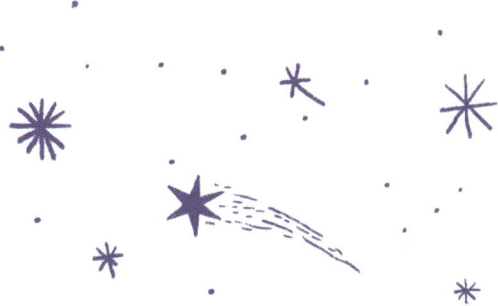

SUPPORTED POSE

Feeling cool and collected starts by looking it, and this casual posture is a great way to start. When presenting to a room, talking to someone you're trying to impress or looking to feel at ease in any situation, it projects relaxed confidence that can turn into genuine calmness and control. And, by physically supporting your body, you'll reduce anxiety and feel more stable.

QUEEN POSE

This posture is reminiscent of how someone regal might sit. It's a posture for someone who knows they are in charge, but is open and welcoming. It's a great option for a seated power pose and establishes authority without being aggressive or domineering. It can trigger your brain to remember who is boss without taking up a huge amount of space (if that's uncomfortable for you) and shows you to be a good listener and friendly expert.

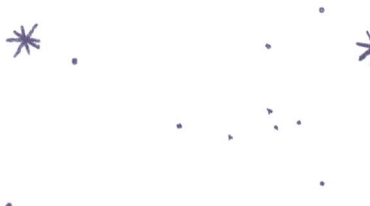

PRESENCE POSE

Physically leaning into a conversation can help with your mental presence, which is why this pose is a great way to be more focused. The extra attention you put on your subject, the less your mind can wander or worry and the more collaborative, calm and confident you'll feel. This is a great one to take when needing to guide a team through a hard decision or negotiation, or when you are committing to learning a new skill that requires you to listen.

ENGAGED LISTENING POSE

There are many reasons why Rodin's *The Thinker* statue draws crowds, and one of them is that it speaks to the philosophical, quizzical nature in humans. Your body may not be sculpted from bronze, but taking on this posture shows signs of intelligence and meaningful thought, giving confidence to those around you while showing that you are deeply considering the discussions. It also gives you space and time to think through the powerful words you'll say.

PERCH POSE

Perching is another way to demonstrate comfort and relaxation. It can show you are so at home in your environment, you are happy to sit or lean on a surface not designed for sitting. This taller, standing posture raises you above your seated colleagues or friends to command attention and, by leaning back on to the table, you'll be maintaining a broad, open posture. This position is the perfect balance of friendly and assertive, just like a true leader.

WHOLENESS POSE

Taking inspiration from one of the most powerful cards in a Tarot deck, wholeness pose is based on The World card. Pulling this card tends to mean you have – or will have – a sense of achievement, fulfilment and completion and is illustrated with a dancing woman. She holds her arms open, ready to accept her winnings, and has a joyful posture with dancing feet and a tilted head, thought to represent her looking back to her past and moving to the future. Holding this pose can help you believe you hold the same wholeness as The World's depicted woman, and may help you develop a sense of lightness and excitement.

CREATIVE POSE

This pose has many benefits for your internal and external perceptions of power and creativity. It's a hip stretch that can tease out stress from the body, and make you feel more comfortable and at ease. A cross-legged position is also shown to stimulate the abdominal muscles, connecting you to your sacral and naval chakra to boost internal fire, creativity and power.

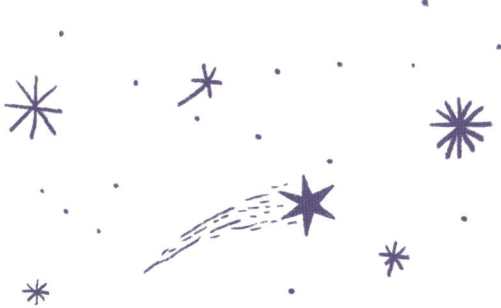

BOX BREATH

Focusing on your breath is a great way to stop your mind from racing when you're feeling anxious, have stage fright or are facing imposter syndrome. Box breathing is a simple, beginner-friendly technique that will help you bring your body and mind out of worry. While it will ease nerves, it's not intensely calming (look at the Resetting Breath card for a fully relaxing breath practice), which makes it great to practise throughout the day – or even mid-conversation – to drop back into a neutral state.

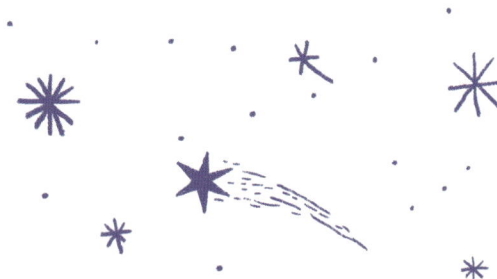

GRATITUDE POSE

It's a mistake to think that showing power or leadership means disrespecting others. In fact, often the most powerful thing you can do is show kindness, appreciation and warmth to others, and having gratitude for those around you is also shown to improve your own self-esteem. Taking hold of your heart centre during difficult conversations – or even easy, lighthearted moments – can improve your connection to yourself and others for an openness you can be grateful for.

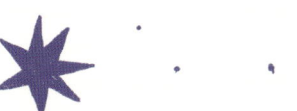

FLOW POSES

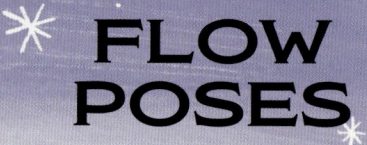

These daily practices work to build
confidence in your body and mind
over time. Use them to destress,
connect with yourself and strengthen
any physical and mental weak spots.

WARRIOR I

Warrior I, known in yoga as Virabhadrasana I, commemorates the Hindu god and mythical warrior Virabhadra, and is a great way to channel your inner power. It's a heroic posture that will help you develop strength in the lower body over time, while also getting you comfortable with holding your body in an expansive and energetic way. Lifting up through your spine, chest, arms and head will open your heart space, which – while vulnerable-feeling to begin with – can lead to powerful breakthroughs in confidence and self-esteem, training you to hold more power in your life outside of the yoga mat.

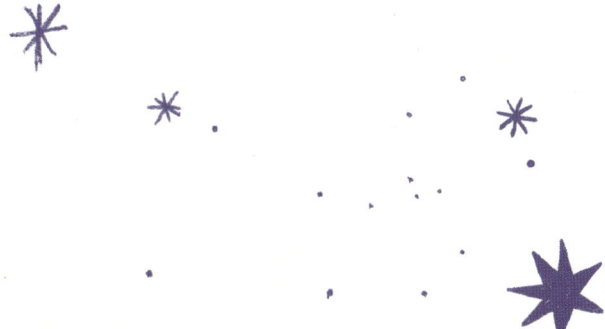

WARRIOR II

Virabhadrasana II is the second pose dedicated to Virabhadra and is a rare posture where you will be strong, grounded, expansive and stretching at once. It's a posture that requires you to take up a lot of space, with your arms extending to their full span and your legs taking a wide position, which is great practice for being big at work, in your relationship or with your social circle. You'll also need to remain focused on the many points of this posture, including how your feet, knees, hips, chest, shoulders and arms align, training you to be more present and less anxious.

WARRIOR III

Virabhadrasana III pose is quite different to the first two Virabhadrasana poses. As a balancing pose, it is much less stable and grounded and much more about finding inner focus and cultivating intense physical strength. You'll improve your ability to balance the expansiveness of the pose with the contraction of your muscles – a delicate act, which requires precision and confidence so you don't topple over, and a brilliantly transferable skill. Practise when you need to prove your inner strength.

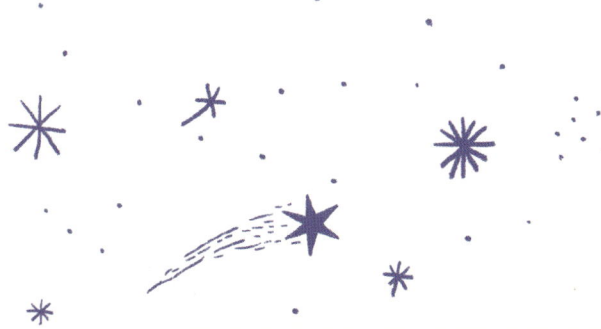

TRIANGLE POSE

A combination of an inversion and standing pose, triangle pose (Trikonasana) can build courage and self-trust. Grounding down through both feet, you'll be energized and stable while expanding the body. Folding forwards challenges your mental and physical balance and your strength while helping to clear your mind by stimulating blood flow. The open arms clear your heart space to build self-love. With continued practise, this pose can be used as proof that you can hold strong and steady, even when the situation feels uncertain or out of balance.

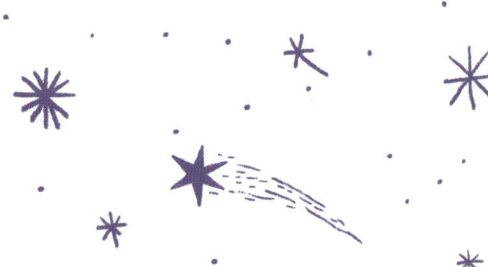

GODDESS POSE

Goddess pose – or Utkata Konasana, which translates to 'fierce angle pose' – is based on the Hindu goddess Kali, who is often depicted as victorious in battle in an open squat position. She is thought to be a representation of divine feminine energy (which all genders have in them), and practising this pose can help you unleash your powerful resilience. The sumo positioning not only takes up physical space but also releases negative energy and stress by stretching out the hips, leaving you feeling positive and self-assured. Holding the arms outstretched in cactus pose will also help you shed fear or worry.

COW FACE POSE

This pose, known as Gomukhasana, requires a lot of attention to alignment, and practising your postural awareness will make it much easier to notice and correct your shrinking body when it matters. While it's a seated, twisted pose, it's also an expansive one, as it opens the upper body and releases tension from the hips. Because of the full-body, deep stretch it gives, it's also a great way to care for your physical self after a long day sat in meetings or at a computer.

TREE POSE

Balancing poses aren't just good for working on your physical stability, but are also useful to harmonize emotions, which is why they can be excellent if you're trying to recalibrate your sense of self. As one of the modern yoga gurus B.K.S. Iyengar once said, 'Balance in the body is the foundation for balance in life.' One of the most loved and simplest balance poses is Vrksasana, or tree pose, as it's adaptable for your skill level and requires grounding, prayer and self-trust – all important for improving sensations of power.

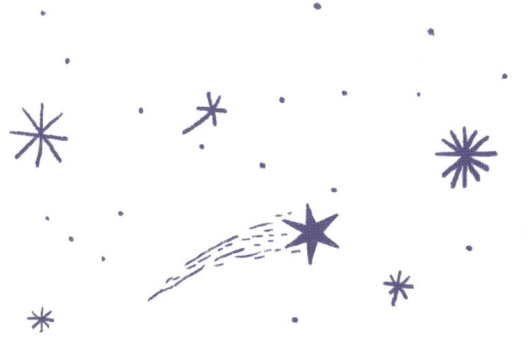

OPEN PALM MEDITATION

In yoga, holding your palms open is thought to help you receive energy, wisdom and blessings from the universe, as well as signal that you're open to growth. Holding this pose while you meditate on your confidence and self-esteem might help stimulate more willingness to develop and call in support in your search for power from forces bigger than you.

CLASPED HAND FORWARD FOLD

Inversions like this are a brilliant way to let go of the day. By placing your heart over your head in clasped hand forward fold, a variation of Uttanasana, fresh clarifying blood rushes to your head and works against gravity to decompress your body and brain. Opening the heart and lowering your head are also thought to balance your body and emotions, dampening the stresses of the day until you're at equilibrium, physically and mentally.

WILD THING

The word 'wild' can be interpreted in many ways, including untamed and out of control. But in this move, also known as Camatkarasana, the word means free-spirited, passionate and miraculous. This pose is the exact opposite position to what our body would do in fear, as it's open, unstable and lacks protection, building your confidence in moments of vulnerability. While this backbend position is a challenging one to find and hold, it's not all serious. Channel the whimsy, delight and carefree expansion in this pose.

SELF-HUG

We know there are plenty of mental and physical benefits to hugging loved ones, but self-hugs are also associated with brilliant outcomes. Giving yourself a hug can improve self-compassion and reduce tension, making it a brilliant way to calm yourself after an intense day. Regular self-touch is also shown to reduce cortisol during stressful moments, meaning you are more resilient, and can improve recovery afterwards. It might feel awkward at first, but you'll soon settle into giving yourself a big squeeze.

DIGESTION POSE

Pawanmuktasana, also known as digestion pose, translates to 'wind removing pose' and is best known for aiding digestion by massaging the ascending and descending colon. With poor digestion being a symptom of a blocked naval chakra, this move can help shift any surrounding negativity for a positive day. Supine poses are also a brilliant way to decompress from hard days and you will feel a relaxing stretch through the front and back of the hips in this pose.

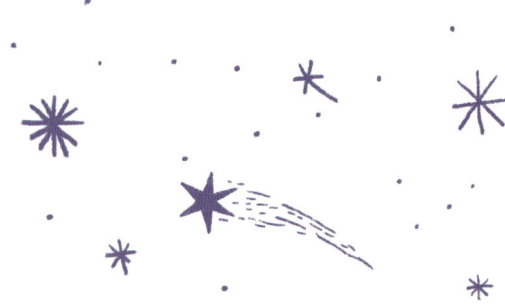

RESETTING BREATH

Any form of exhale-focused, slow breathing will stimulate the vagus nerve, which is responsible for the 'rest and digest' relaxation state. This breathwork practice is rooted in ancient yogic breathing – known as pranayama – and has been developed by Dr Andrew Weil, who calls it a 'natural tranquilizer for the nervous system'. Practise this breath after chaotic days or before bed.

YOGI SQUAT

Malasana, otherwise known as yogi squat, is primarily a hip opener that can aid digestion and reduce tension. However, it's also a position that most of us found natural as a child but which we now struggle to make, and practising it is a brilliant way to come back to our young, carefree and flexible selves. Your range of motion may not be as deep as you see in images of this pose, but it will improve as you find more space in the hips through practice.

HALF PIGEON POSE

Half pigeon – or Ardha Kapotasana – is known to be one of the most effective hip-opening poses in yoga, and it's also great for beginners. Pairing the lower-body, emotional release with a proud, puffed-chest heart opener is a great way to maintain power and confidence during vulnerable moments – a skill you can take off the mat, too.

CRANE POSE

Bakasana, which translates to crane pose, is one of those poses that feels impossible on the first few tries. Then, suddenly, you get it. This posture is a lesson in patient skill development; you get a tiny bit better every time you try until you can nail it. But it also proves that confidence and calmness are equally trainable accomplishments; you'll feel so much more capable in your body the tenth time you try a crane pose versus the first.

LEGS UP THE WALL POSE

The name of this pose may feel too descriptive to be meaningful, but the Sanskrit phrase, Viparita Karani, tells us a lot more about this posture. It translates to 'reversed action', which relates to the changing direction of blood flow for healing and energizing purposes, and also the 'doing nothingness' of the pose. This supported, restorative pose is designed to help calm your nervous system with no over-stretching, hyper-focus or muscle strength required, making it perfect for finding inner peace after busy days.

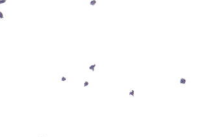

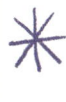

CAMEL POSE

This posture, also known as Ustrasana, is the exact opposite of what we spend the majority of our lives doing. Rather than hunching forwards, it has you leaning back. Rather than biting your tongue, you're opening your throat (where the Vishuddha chakra is located, which is known to improve communication). Rather than feeling weak, you're strong and powerful, with active muscles. Try it when you need a dose of energy and change of pace.

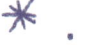

LION'S BREATH

This breathwork looks different from other pranayama (breathwork) practices because it's just as physical as any other yoga asana. Also known as Simhasana pranayama, it's a stimulating, energizing practice that you'll finish feeling powerful and without ego – as you'll have to lean into any silliness you feel when performing this pose – it's also a cleansing posture that will ease restriction in the throat chakra, improving your ability to articulate and express your emotions and needs. That's vital for feeling more confident in your future conversations.

CORPSE POSE

Yoga practitioners believe that corpse pose, known as Savasana, is one of the most important asanas in yoga. It may just look like lying down but there's much more to it than that. Typically performed at the end of a practice (or stressful day), Savasana helps your body move from stimulated to calm, and from fight-or-flight mode to rest-and-digest mode. It keeps the transition between these pathways firing, teaching your body how to down-regulate from anxiety and to be comfortable in stillness. Taking that practice off the mat, you'll be able to hold your ground and self-soothe in difficult situations, leading to a more powerful you.

SEQUENCES

Performing single poses for a few minutes or breaths is enough to re-connect you to your body and mind. But if you want to dive deeper into your power, or simply have more time to play with, then consider adding these sequences – multiple poses practised back-to-back – into your routine. You can get creative with transitions between the postures to find a flow or simply step between them. Each sequence can be done once through, or add more rounds.

✴ **FLOW FOR ENERGY**
1.   Upward Salute
2.   Warrior I
3.   Warrior II
4.   Triangle Pose

✴ **FLOW TO REBALANCE**
1.   Self-Hug
2.   Dynamic Forward Fold
3.   Half Pigeon Pose
4.   Child's Pose

✳ FLOW FOR CONFIDENCE

1. Inner Teacher
2. Prayer Pose With Visualization
3. Open Palm Meditation
4. Lion's Breath

✳ FLOW FOR FOCUS

1. Box Breath
2. Presence Pose
3. Engaged Listening Pose

✳ FLOW TO SOLVE A PROBLEM

1. Standing Thinker Pose
2. Confidence Pose
3. Perch Pose

✳ FLOW TO BOOST CREATIVITY

1. Empowered Pose
2. Creative Pose
3. Lightning Bolt Pose

ABOUT THE AUTHOR AND ILLUSTRATOR

✳ **Chloe Gray** is a fitness instructor and journalist. She writes about women's health, fitness and equality, and is passionate about demystifying exercise and wellbeing.

chloe-gray.com / @graychlo

✳ **Kadna Anda** is a graphic designer and illustrator. She graduated with an MA in Graphic Communication Design from Central Saint Martins, University of Arts London.

kadna.co / @kadnanda

OTHER TITLES IN THIS SERIES

✳ Yoga Asana Cards
✳ Breath Practice Cards
✳ Yoga Through Tarot Cards

Quarto

First published in 2025
by Leaping Hare Press
an imprint of Quarto.
One Triptych Place,
London, SE1 9SH,
United Kingdom
T (0)20 7700 9000
www.Quarto.com

EEA Representation, WTS Tax d.o.o., Žanova ulica 3, 4000
Kranj, Slovenia

ISBN 978-1-83600-367-0
Ebook ISBN 978-1-83600-368-7

10 9 8 7 6 5 4 3 2 1

Editorial: Monica Perdoni, Chloe Murphy
Senior Designer: Renata Latipova
Senior Production Controller: Rohana Yusof

Printed in China